To God,

I can do all things through Christ who strengthens me

To my wife Edypssia,

A Proverbs 31 Woman, and my biggest cheerleader.

To my friends and family,

Your support has meant the world to me.

Table of Contents

Introduction

Are you frustrated with not being able to lose weight? Are you tired of quitting on yourself and others and want to prove to yourself you can lose weight? If you are tired of feeling fat and repeating the same struggles with weight loss, then this book is for you. This book was written with you in mind. This book is meant to give you a breakthrough in your weight loss.

This book was written to help you identify and change aspects of your weight loss approach in a practical way. You don't need theory at this point in your weight loss journey. You need something that will work long term.

This is not a diet book. This is not even an exercise book. There are no shortcuts to fat loss within this book. However, you will learn to avoid the pitfalls that leave you frustrated. By consistently following the success principles in this book, you can begin to change your life. You can begin to increase self-confidence, self-esteem, and self-efficacy.

You are not a failure. Success is in you, but you have to learn how to draw it out. The sooner you come to that realization, the sooner you will achieve your goals. There are no gimmicks in this book, just proven success principles that work if you do the work too. Nothing can hold you back from success in losing weight other than yourself. You can do it. You can have your breakthrough.

But, nothing will change on the scale unless the mind changes first. Don't waste another day looking for the next fad diet. Otherwise, this time next year you will still be overweight and frustrated. Follow the principles and you can have the confidence you want. You can have a life full of energy, health, and joy.

But with any goal, there will be challenges. Within this book are tools to overcome them. Avoiding these 10 mistakes will get you to your goal. Everyone that has successfully lost weight and kept it off has mastered the tools over time. This includes myself. Once I changed my mindset, my body followed. You can have the same success by mastering the following tools and avoiding the 10 major pitfalls to losing weight.

Chapter 1: Going In With the Wrong Mindset

Not having the end in mind

What is your ultimate goal? What is it that you want to accomplish? Where do you see yourself two weeks from now? A month from now? Six months from now? A year from now?

These are important questions to answer. Going into a long-term commitment without a goal is like taking a road trip without a destination. This is a mistake that will inevitably lead to failure. You must challenge yourself to think about attaining your goals in the future.

Forward thinking equals forward progress. It is not good enough to just write your goals down, you need to constantly have them on the front of your mind. Your goals need to be in front of you to remind you of your commitment to yourself. Nowadays, we are bombarded with many different messages throughout our day. This may be from loved ones, TV, social media, work, etc. How many of those messages are motivating you towards your goals?

What you focus on grows and magnifies. Therefore, if you focus and meditate on reaching your goals, they begin to grow and magnify your desire. Meditating on your goals allows the goals you are pursuing to seem more attainable to you. As your desire begins to grow, self-doubt begins to shrink.

Busy people may not have the time to meditate quietly for an extended period of time during the day. But, finding time to take short goal-meditation breaks within your day is beneficial and empowering. This may mean turning off the radio in your car or keeping your TV off once you get home. Perhaps listening to an encouraging podcast, sermon, or audiobook may help you focus on your goals.

But the main thing is keeping your thoughts on your goals. You should display them where you can see them every day, multiple times a day. Begin repeating them out loud thus affirming to yourself that you will get to your goal.

Being okay with trying

Another mistake people make when losing weight is being okay with "trying." Trying is a short term answer for a long term problem. Lasting success can't be built on only short-term efforts. People usually *try things out.* If they don't see results quickly enough, they eventually quit. Weight loss success is not made with that type of mindset. You cannot be okay with trying. To advance in health and fitness, you need to become committed to reaching your goal no matter what.

When one is involved with a weight loss program, a defeatist outlook can manifest. Just trying is like saying: "I will give somewhat of an effort but as soon as it gets too hard I will quit." Or, "I will try until it inconveniences me." Even better, "No one is really expecting me to stick with it anyway; so as soon as I can, I'm quitting". Exercise and eating right is more than just trying—it is a lifestyle. Honestly, when it comes to a weight loss program you have to be ready to change your life and not just your weight.

You cannot enter one of the hardest endeavors of your life with the "try it out" mindset. If so, you are doomed to fail. As you continue to "try" diets only to quit diets, it impacts your self-confidence. Without noticing, you begin to lose confidence in your ability to complete any task, even tasks outside of health and fitness. Your belief in your ability to complete tasks is known as self-efficacy. Having low self-efficacy will begin to erode your self-esteem.

Low self-efficacy causes you to gravitate towards things that require less effort. You will search for easier diets to get results. Unfortunately, you will find out that if it doesn't challenge you, it won't change you.

Making a lifestyle change necessitates commitment, much like marriage, a mortgage, or a college education. You have to think long-term. You cannot sacrifice your long term goals for shortcuts or instant gratification. You have to be willing to endure to reach your goal. If not, you are only setting yourself up to quit.

Storytime: Cosmetic Surgery vs. Exercise

When I was a personal trainer, I met a young lady that was interested in toning and tightening her arms and legs; this was by way of post-cosmetic surgery where she got a "tummy-tuck." She realized after surgery that her arms were abnormally larger than her newly shaped torso. I told her, to achieve her goals, it would take a few months before seeing results, and she agreed to "try" personal training. We began with a free 30-minute session. It was intense but doable. We tried different three arm and three leg machines, completing two sets of 10 repetitions on each machine. Afterward, we agreed to begin training the following week.

Sad to say, I have not seen her since. She already had some "success" taking shortcuts which cemented a quick-result mindset. Honestly, in her mind, she never really wanted to train, just obtain the final results. Her two options were giving exercise a try or pay for another surgery. One required effort and the other one didn't.

She paid a significant amount of money for her new flat stomach. She could've spent the same amount on personal training two times per week for a year and gained self-confidence, strength, and the body she wanted. But her shortcut-mindset was all wrong.

Build slowly

Gradual changes seem to be the best practices for success. Big changes require big efforts. Likewise, small changes require small efforts. Starting off with a maximum effort may be too much of a price to pay at the beginning. Maximum results cannot be attained by paying with minimal effort. This mindset never works. Maximum results have a high price and must be paid upfront.

However, gradual changes are easier to maintain. As you become more consistent, the results will become more apparent. Therefore, setting smaller, more attainable goals and achieving them will build self-efficacy.

Your strengths as resources

Setting goals within your strengths is needed for a successful lifestyle change. Knowing your strengths require that you know yourself. Being honest about your strengths and weaknesses can only help you achieve your goals. This can be scary but must be done. If you are not sure what your strengths are, ask few people you know will be honest with you about your strengths and weaknesses.

Setting goals within your strengths sets you up for victory. For example, if you are a morning person, be a morning person. However, if you are not a morning person, it is okay, but don't promise that you will get up every morning at 5:30 AM to workout. Find a way to workout when you have the most energy in your day. This may be in the evenings or late night.

Moreover, your goals have a price that must be paid in full daily. Every single morning when you wake up, you have to make the decision to pay the price for your goal. If you are operating in areas of weakness, such as not being a morning person but promising to workout in the morning, it may not work long term. The commitment may seem too high of a price to pay that early in the morning. But, it may not seem too high of a price to pay later in the day because you are operating in an area of strength.

Best Practices: Staying committed

To stay committed to your goals, focus on your strengths and begin to set goals within them. For "night owls" or people who find it easier to stay up late, it may mean working out at night. Be sure to stretch and shower afterwards to help you fall asleep after a workout.

Another way to stay committed is making sure that you prepare for your next workout ahead of time. For example, pack your gym bag from the night before. Additionally, keep your gym bag in the same place every time so you don't forget it. Keeping it together with everything you need to take with you to work the next day ensures that you will remember it.

In addition, don't give yourself the opportunity to misstep. Avoid going home from work to prepare for the gym. Once your workday is over, try your best to go straight to the gym. Begin with getting into your workout clothes at work (sneakers and all). While driving, circumvent any streets leading to your house and drive directly to the gym. Listening to something motivational on the way to the gym will help inspire you to workout. Avoid anyone or anything that may distract you. This may mean not starting any telephone conversations or listening to negative things on the radio.

Find your own unique ways to stay committed based on your schedule and strengths. You will be surprised how creative you can be.

Chapter 1: Going In With The Wrong Mindset
Quotes to Live by

"Do or do not. There is no try." – Yoda, Star Wars

"Know yourself to improve yourself." – Auguste Comte

"The new year stands before us, like a chapter in a book, waiting to be written. We can help write that story by setting goals." – Melody Beattie

"Let's not get tired of doing what is good, for at the right time we will reap a harvest—if we do not give up." – Galatians 6:9

"Everything you want in life has a price connected to it. There's a price to pay if you want to make things better, a price to pay just for leaving things as they are, a price for everything." – Harry Browne

Chapter 2: Not Having a Plan

Not planning to succeed is planning to fail. It sounds like a cliché, but most truths are. Going in without a plan is like trying to hit a target on a wall, in the dark, blindfolded, in an airplane hangar. Yes, it is that difficult.

Planning is more than just knowing your goal, writing it down, and keeping it on your mind. You need a realistic plan to attain the goal. Imagine wanting to save $30,000 for a down payment on a house. What would be the first thing you do? What would be the second thing? How long is it going to take you? Where are you going to keep the money? Are you going to do it alone?

These are all important questions. But what is more important is the detail within the answers. Staying broad and general keeps you in the airplane hangar. The lights might be on but you are still blindfolded. The more the detail, the fewer the obstructions you have preventing you from hitting the target. Even if you are at one end of the airplane hangar and your target is all the way at the other end, you can progressively make your way closer to the door. Going too broad ensures that you will hit nothing but planning ensures that you will eventually get close to your goal.

The more detailed the plan, the more successful the plan will be. Just saying I want to lose 25 lbs. in 3 months isn't enough. How do you plan on doing it? Where are you going to work out? What form of exercise are you going to utilize? How are you going to cut calories out of your diet? Answering these questions with detailed answers provides a blueprint for success.

Aiming low and hitting

Setting low goals may cause more harm than good. For example, if someone were planning on losing one pound a week and after 3 weeks they lose only 3 pounds, they would be more disappointed than happy of their accomplishment. There is nothing wrong with losing 3 pounds. I believe it should be celebrated (not with food). But the disappointment of just getting exactly what you worked for can be detrimental.

You get what you work for. But as humans, we expect more than what we worked for. Nevertheless, that is not how losing weight works. Low goals require low efforts. But accomplishing small goals are never enough to boost self-efficacy and self-esteem. However, high goals require high efforts. Much more of an effort than we believe we can give. Only when we are challenged to push past our perceived capacities do we unearth things about ourselves we didn't know we possessed. Through these discoveries, we boost self-efficacy and self-esteem.

Overcoming challenges allows you to find out that there is more in you than you originally thought. The new thoughts about yourself challenges the previous thoughts you had about yourself. Now, when the next challenge comes, you will say "I probably can if I stick to it." This is probably much different than the belief you held against yourself before all, based on the perception you have about your ability to reach a goal.

Therefore, aim high. It is perfectly fine to have high goals if you are willing to pay the price for them in time, effort, and sacrifice. Reaching high goals require that they be broken down into smaller steps.

Storytime: The Chubby Trainer

When I finally decided to take exercise seriously and lose weight, it took a lot of planning and discipline on my part. What prompted the change was after a vacation in Puerto Rico, I saw a few photographs of myself. Truthfully, I didn't even recognize the person in the photos. I was overweight. Back then, my blood pressure was high for an active person in their mid-twenties.

At the time, I was working as a personal trainer. Yes, I was the chubby trainer at the gym. Honestly, I never realized I was that big until seeing the photos. Once I saw them, I knew I had to change. So I made a plan.

Firstly, I assessed my body. I took a hard look at the areas of my body needing improvement and compiled a list. These were the areas I needed to work on first at the gym. I used most of my energy on the worst problem areas and then worked on the others. I hated doing abs, so I made sure that was the first thing I did once at the gym.

Next, I had to improve my diet. I was a notorious late eater. My last meal would be around 11 PM. Late eating caused a lot of weight gain around my stomach. So I started eating earlier and began to see results. Then I added foods that would give me the most energy for my next workout. Thus, I incorporated more fruits and vegetables into my diet. I ate the majority of my carbs in the morning and decreased my carb intake in the afternoon.

I made a plan to workout three days a week on Mondays, Wednesdays, and Fridays. On my days off, I decreased my calorie consumption to avoid gaining weight. I removed sweets from my house and cut fried foods from my diet.

It took time, but I eventually got control of my diet. I started with small changes and built upon them as I began to see results. I started with small changes I could commit to.

Eventually, I lost 45 lbs. in three months. It took planning and sacrifice, but I achieved it. I had to practice what I was preaching. Through my experience I learned many things about myself and the difficulties of losing weight. Now I help others do the same.

From light pole to light pole

All large ventures can be accomplished if you break them down into smaller steps or milestones. With each completed milestone, there is a sense of progress towards the ultimate goal. Focusing on reaching just the next milestone keeps you from feeling overwhelmed. I call this running from light pole to light pole. You can run longer distances than you think if you just focus on reaching the next light pole before you. Once you pass that light pole, focus on reaching the next light pole, then repeat. Before you know it, you are running further than you ever ran before.

Likewise, rather than worrying about losing an entire 100 lbs., focus on losing the first 5-10 lbs. in a month. Just focus on what you have to do to reach the first 5-10 lbs. goal—nothing else. As you reach that goal, focus on the next 5-10 lbs. for the next month. As you move forward, you will begin building self-efficacy and self-confidence to the point that you will begin challenging yourself to reach larger goals within a month.

Therefore, instead of looking at your goal as one large mountain, focus on the small steps to scale the mountain. Whatever you focus on magnifies or becomes. The more we focus on the size of the mountain, the larger the mountain becomes. As a result, our perceived ability to accomplish the goal shrinks. However, if you focus on breaking your large goal into smaller ones, your perceived ability to accomplish them magnifies.

Planning for challenges

The largest misstep in the planning process is the lack of planning for setbacks, obstacles, and difficulties. Each has its own respective issues and should be planned for, accordingly. They are a part of the change process and are coming whether you want them to or not. Great goals are always accompanied by great challenges. The two cannot be separated. Challenges are meant to grow you. It is not possible to be the same person after "growing" through challenges. There are things that only challenges teach you that success can't.

- *Setbacks* are missteps that are made during dieting or exercising that causes someone to quit. This challenge is usually at the initial stage of goal attainment. Setbacks are usually self-inflicted from self-sabotaging habits that were developed from past failures. Most people stop at this stage because they never developed the self-denial or will-power needed to attain a goal. For instance, this can be eating too much at a party or going on vacation and "forgetting" about working out or eating right. Developing the will-power to deny yourself is needed to reach any goal. Thus, when other challenges arise, you can use your will-power to overcome. Your will-power grows each time you choose success over setbacks when you are confronted with a decision. Eventually, if you use your will-power enough, it becomes a habit.

- *Obstacles* are the next stage of the challenges. Obstacles are hindrances that get in the way long enough to discourage you from continuing. The hindrances seem large, immovable and the closer you get to your goal, the larger the obstacles become. For example, plateauing at a certain weight. Regardless of what you do, you can't get past a certain weight. Obstacles are meant to develop your resiliency. You have to endure through the obstacles to overcome it. Eventually, you will surpass the obstacle and grow your self-confidence.

- **Difficulties** are the last stage of the challenges. Difficulties are distractions that arise to stop you just before reaching your goal. The difficulties are usually large enough to require you to solely focus on resolving the distraction. For example, a death of a loved one, car accident or large financial difficulties. The more intense the distraction, the closer you are to your goal. Difficulties are meant to teach you commitment. The distractions seem unbearable, great, and menacing, ready to take you out. Are you going to quit or double-down on your commitment? Overcoming the distraction will require you to take your diet and exercise to another level. You will have to find new creative ways to stay committed to your health and fitness goals while dealing with the distraction too. This requires a greater effort than the first two challenges. You will have to do things you have never thought about doing before to reach your goals. A leap of faith may be necessary to overcome the distraction. But once you overcome the distraction, you would have developed the ability to stay committed regardless of what happens in your life.

Regardless of the challenge, you must plan for them. Don't just plan for the different steps required to achieve your goals but contingencies for when the challenges arise. You may have to increase your workouts or become stricter with your diet. You may need to reach out and get help from others to help you carry the burden and hold you accountable. But once you overcome these challenge, you become unstoppable. You become more than a conqueror. You become an overcomer.

Chapter 2: Not Having a Plan Quotes to Live by

"A goal without a plan is just a wish." – Anonymous

"If it doesn't challenge you, it won't change you." – Anonymous

"Then the LORD replied: "Write down the revelation and make it plain on tablets so that a herald may run with it." – Habakkuk 2:2

"Proper planning prevents poor performance." – Steven Keague

"Ask yourself if what you are doing today is getting you closer to where you want to be tomorrow." – Anonymous

Chapter 3: Going At It Alone

The Lone Ranger?

Even the Lone Ranger had a sidekick. The Lone Ranger is a fictional character who was a former Texas Ranger who fought outlaws in the American Old West with his Native American sidekick, Tonto. Most heroes have sidekicks because they knew sidekicks were needed help to save the day.

The quote "No man is an island" speaks to the difficulty to stand on one's own. But asking for help is not a sign of weakness. It is foolish not to ask for help when you need it. One piece of advice from others will save you time, effort, and money. Do you want to waste time, effort, and money very foolishly?

Honestly, asking for help takes humility and courage. Many people are apprehensive about asking for help because of the negative response they may get from the helper. This couldn't be further from the truth. People are more helpful than you expect. Asking the helper is a form of flattery because you are saying that you value them and what they know. Because of this, many times people will go above and beyond what you asked them for.

The power of accountability

No man is an island. This quote means that no one can stand alone, we all need one another. Help from others makes reaching any goal possible. The greater the goal, the more help you will need.

What I have found is that people set secret goals so if they quit, no one else will know. But, this is a recipe for failure. Not allowing others to know about your goals leaves you to be accountable to yourself. Being accountable to yourself takes a great deal of self-discipline. This characteristic may be underdeveloped if you have failed to hold yourself accountable in the past.

However, allowing others to hold you accountable gives you extra incentive to reach your goals. Knowing that someone is going to ask you about your progress encourages you to get back on task. You don't want to disappoint them. But underutilizing this powerful tool can prevent you from accomplishing your goals. There is power in numbers; therefore, find the right person to help you reach your goals.

A big reason why personal training works is because of the accountability. Knowing someone is holding you accountable to your goals keeps them on the front of your mind. You are less likely to eat certain foods knowing that you will be challenged at your next workout session. You are more likely to get into bed on time knowing that your workout is early in the morning. You are able to hold your bad habits in check when you know that there is a weigh-in at the end of the week.

Storytime: A little coaching goes a long way

A training prospect came to me in tears; this wasn't the first time and with experience, I have learned to allow the trainee to let their emotions go before continuing the conversation. She was frustrated with her lack of success in losing weight. She claimed to have tried everything to reach her 40 lbs weight loss goal but failed. She was working out consistently 4 days out of the week but never saw results. Seeking help was her last resort before giving up altogether.

My question to her was "Why did you wait so long to get help?" She replied, "I thought I would be able to do it on my own." I said, "The only thing you should own is your effort, but everyone needs guidance." I explained how no one could lose weight and keep it off successfully by themselves—support, guidance, and accountability are always needed.

After some questioning, she realized she was keeping her weight loss efforts a secret because of the trials and failures in her past. She didn't want anyone to know if she cheated on her diet or gained weight. Doing it alone caused her many secret failures, but she had no one to encourage or support her through failure. The secret failures only frustrated her, and she would return to a vicious weight loss cycle and gain even more weight.

Eventually, I coached her with some tune-up training sessions when her results plateaued. With guidance, she took on newer and more intense fitness challenges and surprised herself with what she could accomplish. She lost over 25 lbs. and several inches and grew in self-confidence.

Seeking professional help

Humility is acknowledging that you do not know everything, and you can learn from others. However, arrogance is believing that you know everything and there is nothing anyone can teach you. Not asking for help can be a form of arrogance. Truthfully, you can learn from anyone.

Seeking knowledge is seeking the best possible way to get to your goal. When you choose not ask for help you are choosing to struggle. Struggling is not a virtue. Wasting time, effort, and money will burn you out and eventually you will quit.

When it comes to losing weight, seeking advice is one of the wisest things you can do. Many health and fitness professionals have spent years researching and educating themselves on the best practices for losing weight. Many don't have hidden agendas and know what is going to work for the long term.

Approaching a health and fitness professional about your challenges with weight loss can be intimidating. However, what they are able to share with you can ultimately remove some of the hurdles you are currently facing. All you may need is a slight adjustment to see drastic results. This can save you weeks of frustration.

Accountability Partners

Accountability Partners are needed to keep us focused on our goals by encouraging us and reinforcing positive behavior. Their job is not to supervise. This is a partnership meant to help develop personal accountability. Bad habits are the basis of unsuccessful weight loss. It takes purposeful effort to change and overcome them. It is natural to regress into bad habits, therefore changing them requires vigilance. When it becomes difficult for you to keep your promises to yourself, you may need an accountability partner. They can help you recognize where you are falling short and point you in the right direction.

Bad habits can be difficult to overcome, which is the reason why they are easy to fall back into; they are developed over time and it can be difficult to break alone. However, having someone there to coach you along may make the biggest difference between you sticking to your goals or quitting.

Personal Accountability

Todd Herman, Performance Coach to Pro and Olympic athletes, has the great definition for personal accountability: Being willing to answer—to be accountable—for the outcomes resulting from your choices, behaviors, and actions.

Todd Herman goes on to say that simple personal accountability definition focuses on the outcomes, which are at the END of the process. In reality, "personal accountability" encompasses ALL phases of the process—the before, during, and after. Throughout the process, you must be WILLING (not forced) to PERSONALLY take ownership for...

- Understanding and accepting the task.
- Taking actions to achieve agreed-upon results.

- Answering the results obtained, regardless of the outcome.

Accountability is related to the key notion behind accounting—to give an account of:

- What resources were entrusted to you,
- What you did with them, and
- What outcomes you produced.

Therefore, if you have failed in the past losing weight, you must own it. Taking ownership is the first step in losing weight now. Taking responsibility causes a shift in mindset. Now you are empowered because you are in control. You will find strength knowing that no one or nothing can stop you—only you can make the decision to quit. However, learning to hold yourself accountable is something that has to be developed over time.

Developing a Personal Accountability System

Developing a personal check-and-balance system is possible and necessary for long-term weight loss success. But, negative behaviors can't be part of the equation. Positive results don't come from negative behaviors. For example, you cannot eat whatever you want and blame others for the weight gain.

Self-examination should be part of any check-and-balance system. Are you working hard enough for the results you want? Are you doing your best with your current resources? What are you producing with your time, money, and effort? If you are answering no to any of the questions, it is time to change and develop your personal accountability system.

Firstly, you must take personal responsibility for every outcome—good or bad. For example, if you weigh-in overweight, instead of looking for someone to blame, ask yourself, "Was there more I could have done?" At the end of the day, it is your weight to lose and no one else's. Blaming others won't take the weight off.

Second in developing your personal accountability system is being honest with yourself when it comes to your decision making. Where you are now is the result of all the decisions you have made in your past. If you want to change your future, you have to change the decision making. Your decisions brought you here, but it is only your decisions that will bring you out.

Thirdly, learn ways to develop strength in areas of weakness. You should avoid situations that you are weak in until you develop the strength to make better decisions. It is unrealistic to think you can avoid these situations forever.

Therefore, find techniques to strengthen the weakness in the meantime. One of the best ways to develop the strength is to learn from someone with the strength. You never know they might have struggled with the same challenge in their past, but developed the skills necessary to overcome the challenge. They can coach you towards developing your own skills.

The fourth and final step to developing a personal accountability system is putting to practice what you have learned. If you want to lose weight, you have to practice developing your skills until you master them. It is not about being perfect but making progress. There may be missteps along the way, but it is about learning from them and getting better from the experience.

Chapter 3: Going At It Alone Quotes to Live by

"But I tell you that everyone will have to give account on the Day of Judgment for every empty word they have spoken." – Matt. 12: 36

"It starts with you." – Anonymous

"Accountability is not what we do, but what we do not do, for which we were accountable." – Moliere

"The only mistake you can make is not asking for help." – Sandeep Jauhur

"Be strong enough to stand alone, smart enough to know you need help, and brave enough to ask for it." – Anonymous

Chapter 4: Choosing the Wrong Help

Sinking boats

The last chapter we made it clear that you need help to achieve anything great. Losing weight is a journey and you need a team of people to keep you accountable, encouraged, and focused. However, having the wrong help can be detrimental to your progress. Having the wrong people helping you becomes more of a burden than help.

I have a saying that "if your boat is sinking and your friend's boat is sinking, then you can't help each other." This means that because you two have not mastered the necessary skills for success, currently you too are unable to help each other. Because of the lack of mastery, your partnership in the weight loss endeavor becomes a Dependent-Dependent Partnership. Ultimately, the goal is to have an Independent-Independent Partnership for success.

I consider them partnerships because they are two parties that join together with each contributing for the expected end of success in a certain endeavor. This is different than a relationship where two parties share a common interest, habits and may or may not have a common goal. In a Dependent-Dependent Partnership, each individual has little or nothing to contribute. Each person is looking to the other to push them to their weight loss goal. These relationships ultimately fail because one of the parties quits, and then the other quits from carrying two burdens instead of their own.

However, losing weight is a learning experience. There are negative habits that need to be unlearned and positive habits that need to be adopted. Therefore an Independent-Independent is the ideal partnership because both parties have skills to contribute to accomplishing a goal. This partnership shares a common goal, but each party can teach, encourage, or coach each other to develop skills that they may lack to reach their goals. But what makes them Independent-Independent is that they don't solely rely on each other to pursue their goals. They were already pursuing their weight loss goals and had success in doing so. Thus, they would be pursuing their goals regardless of any particular partnership; however, they use the partnership as a means of accomplishing more through accountability, encouragement, and shared learning. But as Independent-Independent, if one party learns something beneficial, they share it with their partner so they can get more results. It becomes two people's boats are heading in the same direction rather than one pulling the other.

For success, you need to partner with someone who has already had success in weight loss, thus creating an Independent-Dependent Partnership. Initially, your partnership will be Independent-Dependent, but you should be transitioning to Independent-Independent. In this partnership, the Dependent party should be learning how to become Independent. The Independent partner is the "Tug Boat" teaching the "Sinking Ship" the skills necessary to become Independent.

This relationship should be growing and evolving as the Dependent partner grows and evolves. However, this is impossible to accomplish in a Dependent-Dependent partnership. Because where one is weak, the other should be strong and coaching the other to strengthen their weaknesses. But, if you both have the same weaknesses, how are they supposed to teach and hold the other accountable? If one falls to a weakness, it will give the other a reason to do the same. For example, if both parties are depending on each other as encouragement to go to the gym. As soon as one begins missing gym days on a continual basis, eventually the other will stop going.

This is different in an Independent-Dependent and Independent-Independent partnership. In an Independent-Dependent relationship, if the Dependent partner begins to miss gym appointments, the Independent partner will hold the other accountable. The Independent partner will continue to workout and eat well even without the Dependent partner. But, will the Dependent partner continue to workout and eat well on their own? Most likely not. The Dependent partner will regress back into negative behaviors because they did not spend enough time developing the positive behaviors to change.

As the Dependent partner develops the necessary skills for success and can hold themselves accountable, the partnership evolves into an Independent-Independent partnership.

Power of Influence

You are the average weight of the five people you associate the most. This is true because we influence each other without even knowing it. For example, if you are around a new group of people, unknowingly you will begin changing the way that you speak and behave to be able to communicate and relate better with this new group. The more time spent with a new group, the more influence they will have on behavior. The changes are subtle at first but over time become more pronounced. People within the new group may not notice the change, but people in the old group will notice the change within the person. The new group has the power to change your behavior and speech so much that others in your old group will notice.

Moreover, because of influence, beliefs and attitudes will change being around a new group. In time, thought patterns change as thinking conforms more to the thought patterns of the new group. Eventually, no forethought is needed before action and speech because the mind was transformed to think the way the new group thinks. This is most noticeable in the way time and money are spent.

For example, if your new friends watch a lot of reality shows and that is the main topic of discussion among the group, you will begin watching more reality shows, too, so you are able to relate more to the group. If this is true with negative behaviors, the same is true with positive behaviors.

The people you are around the most have the power to influence you negatively or positively. This is why the saying "birds of a feather flock together" is true. The new group has the power to change the way you think, speak, act, and spend your time and money.

Therefore, if you are overweight, and all of your friends are overweight, you will most likely stay overweight. However, if you find a new group of healthy and active friends, you will become healthier and more active by the power of influence. You will begin thinking, speaking, and behaving like a healthier person. You begin spending time and money on things that make you healthier, and less time and money on unhealthy habits.

Truthfully, changing unhealthy habits into healthy habits becomes difficult if you are around people with unhealthy habits. It is more difficult to change the culture of the group than finding a new group because positive habits cannot be supported by a negative culture. Bishop Tudor Bismark once said, "If you place a good apple among rotten apples, the good apple will become rotten." Just because an apple is good, it cannot change rotten apples around it into good apples. You may have a history with the old group of unhealthy people, but you will not have much of a future with them. What you see in them now is tied to the future you will have with them.

Storytime: Growing and Losing

I had the pleasure of meeting a young lady who successfully lost 80 lbs. in 18 months. During our coaching session, we discussed some of her successes during the last year-and-a-half. When she was overweight, she suffered from low self-esteem and self-confidence. In addition, her friends were overweight, too, and later learned that their expectations limited her expectations for herself.

Once she decided to lose weight, she invited her friends to join her. They began as a large group working out together and trying to hold each other accountable with their diets. Nevertheless, the group got smaller over time. Many of her friends made excuses and expected her to skip workouts on the days when they couldn't make it. She did at first but realized it was her goals she was skipping out on and not her friends. If she wanted her goals, she had to own them. Hence, she recommitted herself and began going to gym regardless if her friends went or not.

After a few months, her friends started noticing the change in her both physically and mentally. Perhaps, unintentionally, they began sabotaging her efforts. They would plan gatherings on evenings they knew she worked out, but per her commitment, she would meet up with them after the gym. Also, her friends would only have get-togethers involving high-calorie foods that they swore to abstain from months earlier. But per her commitment, she stuck to ordering healthier portion-controlled entrees from the menu. Additionally, the group conversations always seemed to be negative. She never noticed before but as her inner conversations changed, she realized her outward conversations needed to change, too. Thus, she spent more time listening than participating in negative talk.

The more time she spent away from her friends, the more her perception changed about herself and other aspects of her life. Over time, she realized that she was growing her friends were not. They were content to stay where they were; she was fighting to move on. Eventually, she lost those friends but gained self-confidence and self-esteem as she got closer and closer to her weight loss goal. Losing the 80 lbs. was a large accomplishment in her life but the person she became along the journey was even more important.

Finding an Elevated Group

In the personal development industry, it is said that if you are the smartest person in your group, you need to find a new group. What this means is if you want to grow as a person, you have to surround yourself with people better off than you. Being in an elevated culture will grow and stretch you. The new elevated group can teach you and introduce you to newer opportunities to stretch your imagination. What you couldn't conceive in your mind before becomes the norm in an elevated group. Therefore, as a man thinks thus is he.

Finding an elevated group is imperative for growth and success. To find an elevated group, you must first be clear on what you want. Do you want comfort or growth? You cannot have both! Not being clear on what you want will cause you to waiver between what you want more of and what you already possess. If you desire to change your life, you have to be clear that you want to lose weight. You can't behave in a way that contradicts what you want. What are your actions saying about your desires? You cannot spend time and money on things that will not bring you closer to your weight goal.

Secondly, you have to be honest about your weaknesses. You cannot change a problem if you deny that there is a problem. Be honest with yourself and be open to receiving help from others to develop your weaknesses. Remember the elevated group has experienced and is living what you want, they will be the best people to advise you on how to grow from where you are.

Thirdly, find a group of people that practice a healthy lifestyle. They must practice a healthy lifestyle to be considered in the elevated group. They cannot talk the talk and not walk the walk. If not, this can be harmful to your development because you are not learning how to replace negative habits with positive ones. Rather look for a group that has strengths in areas that you are weak in.

To find these groups, you have to be where these groups congregate. There are plenty Meetup groups that have a healthy purpose. Additionally, you may find these groups at 5K races, or a local fitness studio. Wherever they are is where you need to be. When you are around them, don't be afraid to ask questions about health and fitness. And follow through on the advice and report back to the advisor. People are always willing to give advice to those they feel will utilize it.

Avoiding Sabotage

However, there are groups of people that cannot be avoided such as your family members, co-workers, and spouses, etc. There is no choice but to interact with them on a daily basis. Because they cannot be avoided, you may be subject to their beliefs, attitudes, and behaviors for a majority of your day. These unavoidable groups tend to have an influence on your weight loss success because of the principle that you become more like the people you associate with the most.

Since you spend the most time with these individuals, these relationships are important. They should be supporting you during your lifestyle change. But they may not share your new beliefs, attitudes, and action and will present pushback because of the change. The pushback may be subtle, but it is meant to sabotage your efforts. They may be unaware that they are sabotaging, but the effect is still the same.

If your family is full of overweight overeaters, most likely that is where you formed your negative eating habits. Your family may be accustomed to eating unhealthy and overeating and may not be receptive to changing the way they eat. You will be presented with opposition when you tell them that you are changing your negative eating habits. There will be pushback because no one wants to be seen as being wrong. People will associate with others who have similar negative behaviors because they won't be confronted about their negative behaviors and won't be asked to change. For this reason, they will not support you and will try to sabotage your efforts.

To avoid familial sabotage will take a great effort. You will have to limit your time around family functions dealing with food and alcohol. Know that there is a possibility of falling back into negative habits when you are around them. Therefore, you must prepare yourself for being in that environment. One way is to eat healthy before the family event thus limiting the amount of calories you can consume with your family. Another way is to make sure that you always have your hands full; that way, no one can hand you another plate of food.

Avoiding sabotage at work is similar to your family. You really don't get to choose who you work with, therefore you are subject to being around negative influences. But coworkers might be more receptive than your family will about your healthy lifestyle change. However, if your coworkers are not, there are ways to avoid their negative behavior. If possible, try exercising before work. You are less likely to make mistakes throughout the day if you begin your day right.

Another way is trying to eat lunch alone by waiting to eat your lunch after everyone has already taken a lunch. Additionally, try keeping water at your workstation and drink throughout the day. This will keep you full and less likely to snack on anything unhealthy. There are apps on your smartphone that you can set reminders on when to drink water.

Some other pitfalls to avoid are afterwork events at bars or restaurants. Always remember that the calories from alcohol and restaurant food add up exponentially. The restaurants may not have healthier options for you, which can easily set you up to eat unhealthy because of the circumstances.

Sabotage from a spouse is the most common form of unavoidable sabotage. Most spouses don't realize that they are sabotaging your weight loss efforts. But their motivation may come from unconscious feelings of worry that if you get fit and healthy, you will leave them. This is untrue, but this unconscious motivation keeps them from supporting your workout and healthy eating efforts in order for you to stay with them. This happens more with a spouse that is unwilling to make the change with you thus you will be met with resistance. To avoid it, you may have to rearrange your schedule significantly to be able to balance all of your responsibilities plus working out and eating right. You may have to get up early, and workout before anyone gets up and be back in time to handle other responsibilities. You may have to prepare two types of food, one for your spouse and one healthier option for yourself. But under no circumstance do you fold under the pressure and give up on your dreams of being healthy.

Spousal sabotage is the biggest detriment to your success because instead of supporting your changes and sharing family responsibilities, they usually work against you until you quit. It is sad but true. That is why it is important to find the right group of supporters as soon as possible. They can support you during the transition. You may be able to find healthy "Meetup" groups on the internet or join running or cycling clubs. Most importantly, find a group of people who practice the healthy lifestyle you want. Your future success depends on it.

Chapter 4: Choosing the Wrong Help Quotes to Live by

"What surrounds us is what is in us." – T.F. Hodge

"Is the company you keep keeping you back?" – Jarod Kintz

"Do two people walk hand in hand if they aren't going to the same place?" – Amos 3:3

"You become like the 5 people you spend the most time with. Choose carefully." – Anonymous

"People inspire you, or they drain you- pick them wisely." – Hans F. Hansen

Chapter 5: Not Doing Your Research

Everyone is unique

There are no two people on the planet that are exactly alike. Even identical twins have different fingerprints and personalities. Because we are all unique, there cannot be a one-size-fits-all approach to your health and fitness goals. In the fitness industry, there are general rules that may apply to a large part of the population; however, there are many exceptions to every rule.

One of the worst misinterpreted tools of the fitness industry is the Height vs. Weight Chart. These charts are supposed to give you a general weight range according to your height. However, the misinterpretation occurs when most people believe that they should be a certain weight for their height according to the chart.

Most of these Height vs. Weight charts don't take into consideration the different body types, and combination of body types, races, bone density difference, etc., that we have on the planet.

For example, thin-frame vs. medium-frame vs. big-frame. Additionally, there are the apple-shaped vs. pear-shaped vs. straight-shaped. Also, there are different types of bone structures that allow people to carry muscle-weight and fat-weight differently.

All of this is important when trying to understand the proper weight for your body type. Even more important, understanding that you are unique changes the way that you approach trying to lose weight.

Storytime: Huge differences even though people ate the same foods

Do we all respond to eating tomatoes in the same way? Or any food for that matter?

There was a study reported on the CBS News website in November 2015 that explains unique findings by the researchers. The study was conducted by the Weizman Institute of Science in Rehovot, Israel. What they found through the study was astonishing. There was a sizeable difference in the way participant's bodies responded after eating the exact same foods.

The study was conducted using 800 participants over a week. Data was collected for the blood glucose levels of each participant after eating identical meals throughout the week.

All the participants wore glucose monitors and entered what they ate using a mobile app. The data collected comprised 46,900 meals eaten during the week. Blood glucose levels are important indicators because elevated blood glucose levels are a major risk factor for diabetes and obesity.

One particular participant said that she has struggled losing weight. She has failed at many diets and is now obese and prediabetic. Researchers noticed there was a significant spike in her blood glucose levels each time she ate tomatoes. In this case, her healthy eating may have contributed to her lack of weight loss.

One of the researchers said that finding an individualized, tailored diet for this participant was vital. Some foods in her diet are not typically considered healthy, but would be healthy for her.

Not everything works for everyone. We are all unique.

Believing what you see on television

Don't believe everything that you see on television. You may see many weight loss products accompanied by success stories advertised on television, but remember they are trying to sell you something. One of my favorite sayings is "don't believe the used car salesman." Remember the used car salesman is trying to sell you a car, he may not know everything about the car but enough to sell you. Therefore, when you see weight loss products sold on TV, remember that they are not telling you everything but just enough to sell you. Most weight loss products on the market suggest that you eat well and exercise for maximum results. But the way it may be advertised may lead you to think that it is a miracle pill with no effort needed for success. Hence, the reason for doing your own research. In years past, you really didn't have a choice but to believe the salesman, but with the advent of the internet, you can research anything.

However, if you do enough research on any subject, you will find arguments for and against a particular weight loss belief. For example, exercising on an empty stomach early in the morning. You will find studies that say that it detrimental to your workout and results, but there are studies that say it will help boost metabolism and burn more fat. Yet you will find people that are getting results either way, mostly because they have found what is true for their unique bodies.

Too quick to try things out and then too quick to quit

We all know people that jump from one diet plan to the next. It seems like they are on something new every week. They are too quick to try new things without allowing their bodies to make changes and see results. These types of people are never satisfied and are looking for quick fixes.

48

Quick-fix people are looking for something easier to do that doesn't require them to change their lifestyle significantly. Quick fixes don't last in health and fitness, only eating well and exercising continues to be true over time. But quick-fixes may work only in the short term, then the person usually gains the weight back and more.

A healthy diet and exercise are the immovable pillars of weight loss success. There may be newer ways to diet and exercise but what is true for weight loss is burning more calories than what is consumed. However, there are certain television shows that use their credibility and influence to push products on people who are desperate for change. Unfortunately, the host of these shows may not believe in the particular product themselves, but they are paid to do a job. It doesn't make them bad, but understand that they are being paid well to be the "used car salesman."

So after viewing these shows, people flood into health food stores looking for the new secret to weight loss. They may see some results, but unless they are willing to change their lifestyle drastically, it won't work. They will only frustrate themselves because they were expecting to lose 20 lbs. with no effort but only lose 2 lbs. with the new product. What they don't understand is that these are supplements that are meant to aid in weight loss. Only with proper diet and exercise can maximum results be realized. Results don't just happen. You need discipline over time to see results.

Do your own research

Therefore, do your own research. Not just on the internet but you must experiment by trying new things and taking the time to see what works for you. Not everything on the shelf is going to work for you. Not all diets or all forms of exercise will work for you either. Everyone is unique, so it takes time and trials to truly see what works for you.

If you want to see real weight loss, then get to know your body. Become your own scientist and begin researching yourself. This takes discipline. This takes time. This takes effort. Firstly, you will need to find a way to record everything that you do and eat. This means that you have to record every meal that you eat and the time of day. Additionally, you have to record the workouts that you do and the time of day you do them. It is also important to record the amount of sleep that you get. If you are not getting enough sleep, this will prevent you from losing weight. Not everyone needs the same amount of sleep. Find out how much sleep you need to feel well-rested when you wake up. Then try your best to get that same amount of sleep every night. And as you workout more, you will need less sleep as your body becomes more efficient at utilizing energy.

All this may sound tedious—and it is. However, you will begin seeing patterns in your behavior that may be harmful or helpful with your weight loss. With several weeks compiled, you will see that you may have lost more weight in certain weeks than in others. For weight loss success, take your most successful week and repeat it to see if you can get similar results. If so, then repeat again and again until it stops working.

Once the results stop, find a new way to tweak your week. This means you may have to change the intensity of your workout or cut out a couple hundred calories in your diet. You can cut calories out of your diet by finding creative substitutes for certain high-calorie foods in your diets. Moreover, shifting meal times to earlier in the day may make a significant difference. This is true with moving your last meal of the day to earlier in the evening. Try it out at a certain time of the day for a week and see what results you get. Then move it earlier the next week to see if you get different results.

What is important is that you are trying new things, giving it time to work, and recording the results. You have to take responsibility for your own success. You have to be methodical with your approach. But with each step, you are becoming your own researcher and gaining the knowledge and discipline necessary for weight loss.

Chapter 5: Not Doing Your Research Quotes to Live by

"Don't trust the used car salesman, do your own research." – Gladimir Simeon

"My people are destroyed for lack of knowledge; because you have rejected knowledge, I reject you from being a priest to me. And since you have forgotten the law of your God, I also will forget your children." – Hosea 4: 6

"Always remember that you are absolutely unique. Just like everyone else." – Margaret Mead

"It's always too early to quit." – Norman Vincent Peale

"You can't rush something you want to last forever." – Anonymous

Chapter 6: Inconsistent Home Workouts

It Takes Discipline

Not everyone has the self-discipline needed to workout at home consistently. It takes tremendous discipline to be able to workout in a place intended for rest and family time. Most of our days are spent out making a living, and then we return home to recharge for the next day. But the place meant for rest and recharge must become a place for sweat and effort. Changing this paradigm in the mind for exercise is difficult, but possible.

There is a small percentage of our population that workout at home on a consistent basis. They get up everyday and workout in the designated area in their homes. They work out during the least distracting time in their day to avoid missing their workout. They get up and go to bed at the same time every day to ensure that they will have the energy to workout the next day. They are consistent with their exercise because they are consistent with other parts of their lives to guarantee that they will be able to workout.

Yet, there are others that mean to workout at home daily but fall short. They purchased large, bulky workout equipment with intentions of staying consistent, but do not. They go to bed at different times every night meaning to wake up early the next day to exercise, but do not. Then they try working out later in the day when distractions are at their highest and are unable to complete their workouts. They are inconsistent with exercise because they are inconsistent with other parts of their lives that will help them exercise. Eventually, the large bulky equipment becomes an expensive clothing rack, and all the workout DVDs begin collecting dust.

Consistency through consistency

Therefore, staying consistent with home workouts requires more than just exercise. There are other factors that are involved outside of exercise. Being consistent with these other factors allows consistency with home workouts. Unswerving behaviors will form a routine that you can expect reliable results. But, inconsistent behavior will result in unpredictable results. Going to bed at the same time every night ensures that you wake up well-rested for your workout the next day. Eating healthy foods consistently safeguards that you will have the energy needed to workout. Working out during low-distraction times of the day guarantees that you are not interrupted during your workouts.

However, approaching your sleep, eating and workouts haphazardly guarantees that your results will be inconsistent and perhaps non-existent. Not getting any results usually causes discouragement and people quitting their health and fitness program.

The need for self-discipline

Self-discipline is doing what you don't feel like doing when you are supposed to do it. This includes when you are tired, under the weather, bored, or just feeling lazy. It is easy to have self-discipline when everything is going well—you are getting plenty of sleep and eating well, and no one intrudes on your personal time. But self-discipline is developed when it is challenged. It is when you have the opportunity to not follow-through, but you do anyway. These experiences develop your self-discipline, tenacity, and self-confidence.

But, these days there are more people with their hands on your time than ever before. You may have less time for yourself. This is unhealthy and means that you are too busy and need to find a balance before you get sick. Find the time to be healthy otherwise, your body will begin telling you it needs rest through symptoms. If you are always pouring out your energy for others and not spending time refueling, your body will pay for it. You will have symptoms like chronic fatigue despite the amount of sleep or caffeine you may drink. You will have less patience and be irritable with others. However, when you spend time refueling and recharging, your body benefits. This may require that you escape and go elsewhere so you can recharge.

Storytime: Up before responsibilities

A mother of two started a workout regimen at home using a popular home workout DVD program. Her two kids were of elementary school age and needed her attention from the time they woke up until bedtime. This really limited her time throughout the day to workout.

She had no issues previously when working out at a gym because she would take the children with her and drop them off at the gym's childcare. But now that she was working out at home, she found it hard to create workout space within her family's living space. When she tried working out in the afternoon, her kids would try doing the Workout DVDs with her. This became more of a distraction than a workout. She found herself watching them so they wouldn't get hurt.

Then she tried working out at night after her kids were in bed. But at the end of a long day, she couldn't find the energy to push herself to achieve maximum results. As a result, she decided to workout early in the morning before her family woke up. She began working out at 4 AM at home in her living room. It was tough at first but after a week, her body adjusted and she never looked back.

Since the change in schedule, she found she had more energy and focus throughout the day. She was able to start tending to household chores earlier and finished before her family woke up. She was able to start her day energized and able to give more of herself to her family.

Time away is important

Finding a place that you are comfortable going for an hour out of your day to recharge is important for you both physically and mentally. This may be a gym, but it can also be the park or a fitness studio. Wherever it is, the time away from home responsibilities will refuel you and give you separation between your "me-time" and home.

You will find once you do have a separation, and are disciplined to stick to a routine, you will have more peace and energy throughout. Giving yourself a break from others allows you to be your best self when you are with them.

Best practice for consistency

However, if you are planning on working out at home, here are some best practices. First, you want to make sure you have a designated area just for working out. This is separate from your bedroom, living room, or garage. Having a designated place in your house allows you to separate your resting place from your workout/recharging space.

Second, the workout place needs to be devoid of distractions. This means that you cannot have a phone, food, or family within the space. All these things have the potential to be a distraction and keep you from exercising.

Third is finding a designated time to workout. The best time is early in the morning or late at night when everyone is asleep. But you have to choose the best time for you or when you feel most energized. Some people are morning people and have the most energy early in the mornings thus they should wake up earlier and workout. Others are night owls who are able to workout at late in the evening or at night without it affecting their sleep.

Fourth, everyone needs to know that you have a designated workout place and time. You must stress the importance of you getting your time to workout. Let them know that you need their help keeping your schedule too.

Kids are good at reminding you of things you said you were going to do.

Fifth, try involving your exercise time with family time by keeping your family active. Walking around the neighborhood with your family can be time well spent. Taking the kids to the park and exercising while they are playing can be a way of getting a workout in.

Finally, start with the basics. Only spend money gradually as you are getting more consistent with your workouts. Spending a lot on the front-end without the self-discipline and consistency in place is like buying four brand new tires, and you don't even own a car. By making purchases gradually you will be rewarding yourself for your efforts rather than wasting money.

Chapter 6: Inconsistent Home Workouts Quotes to Live by

"A lack of consistency can bring a lack of interest." – Anonymous

"Training gives us an outlet for suppressed energies created by stress and thus tones the spirit just as exercise conditions the body." – Arnold Schwarzenegger

"Therefore, my beloved brothers, be steadfast, immovable, always abounding in the work of the Lord, knowing that in the Lord your labor is not in vain." – 1 Corinthians 15:58

"With self-discipline most anything is possible." – Theodore Roosevelt

"Discipline is just choosing between what you want now and what you want most." – Anonymous

Chapter 7: Not Scheduling Time to Workout

If losing weight is the most important thing to you, it must be a priority that is proven by your actions. This is reflected on how you schedule your day. Usually, the most important thing takes priority and is done first, the next most important is second, and the least important thing is done last. However, this is not true for most people who have failed at losing weight. Losing weight should be the most important thing for them but they leave it at the bottom of their Daily To-do Lists. They utilize their time and energy accomplishing other goals for the day but leave exercise and preparing healthy meals for when they have the least amount of time and energy.

Excuses over health

Losing weight takes more effort than just deciding—it takes planning. People who have failed at losing weight in the past usually begin well and are consistent until something happens. This can be a sickness, family issues, work issues, etc. Then the issue eventually bumps losing weight off the top of the list. Then they stop exercising and dieting completely. The reasons to focus on the issue may be legitimate, but it can become an excuse if there is no plan to return to the healthy routine.

Moreover, instead of focusing on why you should find a way to stay healthy, we focus on the issues. Instead of adjusting our schedules to stay fit, we allow the issue to grow into an excuse. Now, we say that we are too busy when the truth is we can find time if we really looked for one. The issues may be imperative and authentic, but what can be more imperative than your health?

It is unfortunate that it takes a bad doctor's report for health to become a priority. Many things take precedence until you are too sick to do them. You cannot be there for your loved ones if you are ill. You cannot work and make a living if you are ill. You cannot enjoy life if you are ill. But, it usually takes a bad diagnosis for people to focus on their health. Don't wait until it's too late to do something about it.

Reasons become excuses if they stop you from exercising and eating well. We have to learn to deal with the issues of life but remain steadfast on our goals. Distractions will always come when you are on the path towards a desired goal. It is only a matter of time. But you must plan for these and adjust your daily schedule to fit in time for yourself. Don't allow the issues of life to become hindrances to your goal.

Storytime: Health vs. Work

These days it seems that people are busier than any time before. We seemed to be slaves to our schedules. And we end each day unable to sleep because we forgot that one thing on our to-do list. I met a young lady that was "too busy" to focus on her health. She was working multiple jobs counseling people on self-care but wasn't practicing self-care herself. Working 16-hour days was taking a toll on her body. She began developing health issues that she needed to take medication for.

When we met for a fitness consultation, she could not see herself finding time in her busy schedule to workout. I told her that she had time, but she should schedule her workouts first, then her work-life around her workouts. I believe the statement probably offended her because I didn't see her until almost a year later.

By then her health got worse and she finally decided she was ready for a change. She had goals of getting off the medication, losing weight, and getting pregnant. She began slowly with scheduling her evening private clients around her fitness class schedule. As she lost weight and inches, she began taking morning classes too. This was major because it meant that she was taking more time off of work.

Her workouts became her priority because of how it positively spilled over into other aspects of her life. She had more energy throughout the day which benefited her clients and her husband.

In time, she got off of her medication. She lost so much weight she was able to get pregnant. She and her husband couldn't be happier.

It took time but she eventually learned to prioritize what was important. She learned that starting with your workout first and scheduling everything else second really works. It is the only way to find time when you think you have none.

Contingency Plan

You have to plan to combat when dilemmas happen. Feeling overwhelmed by the issues of life is typical. However, expecting them not to happen will increase feeling overwhelmed. Don't be caught off-guard; plan for the issues. Creating a contingency plan can ensure your fitness success. This means if you are met with a life issue, you have a plan to adapt and stay on course. Your workout schedule may be thrown off a little but you have a plan in place to deal with the stress, time management issues, and other responsibilities.

Having a plan in place will limit the amount of stress that life complications may bring. Having a plan increases your feeling of control, even if it is over just a small portion of your life. By sticking to your plan and overcoming the obstacles, you can increase your self-esteem and self-confidence. The next time you are met by any opposition, you will be able to face it positively.

Therefore, look at your current schedule and see where you could fit in a workout if you needed to. This can be earlier in the morning, on a lunch break, or on the weekends. You may have to think of creative ways of staying active based on your individual schedule.

Finding healthy food alternatives are imperative to staying fit during difficult times. Packing healthy foods for the day may not work with your schedule, but you can still make the effort in finding different ways to fuel your body. Sometimes it's easier to pick up something healthy to eat rather than finding the time to cook. Begin looking for healthy restaurants around your job, your kid's activities or even around your home. But the most important thing is to have a plan, then work your plan.

Best Practices: Power of the schedule

One way to prevent the issues of life from becoming hindrances to your goals are to schedule your workouts first before scheduling anything else in your day. You cannot leave this to chance because chances are it won't get done. Write it into your daily schedule. This can be a written or electronic. Once you have it in your daily schedule then you can begin filling in the rest of your day. This is a great habit to build consistent success.

Additionally, set reminders in your mobile device to help keep your goals on the front of your mind. Set alarms for 2-3 hours to snack, hydrate, and to get up and move. The constant reminders are good for developing a healthy lifestyle mindset.

Best Practices: Meal Shopping and Prep

Moreover, try keeping your meal prep at the same time each day. Also, try scheduling all your shopping the same day of the week to enhance time management. Shop with a list. The list should be built with healthy meal planning in mind. Sticking to your Meal Plan Shopping List will keep cost down by avoiding wasteful spending from impulse shopping. Save lots of time by meal prepping the same day as your shopping. Pack all your healthy snacks and meals for the week ahead as you are unpacking the groceries. If possible, have family help put away groceries while you pack meals and snacks for the week to save time.

Best Practices: Seeing Deadlines

No schedule is complete without deadlines. Including dates to reach your goals on a calendar is imperative to success. Deadlines must be visible to keep it on the front of your mind. Keeping your goals and deadlines visible may keep you from making any dietary missteps. It is a constant reminder to make better choices.

Seeing your goals in front of you on a regular basis commissions your subconscious part of the mind to help you attain the goal. Habits are hardwired within the subconscious mind. Your subconscious mind is constantly looking to help you become more efficient at whatever you are doing. That is why performing any behavior over a 21-day period becomes a habit. That is why you wake up right before your alarm goes off or get that "missing something" feeling when your break your routine.

Therefore, healthy habits will grow over time by recruiting the subconscious. Eventually, fewer reminders are needed to eat well, drink water, and get active. Soon you will begin waking up before your alarm goes off. It will be easier to begin your day with healthy habits until it's second nature.

With each growing healthy habit, you get closer to reaching your goals. Deadlines become less frightful and become more attainable as you get closer. Begin making strides towards your goals each day by scheduling your workouts, meal prep, and deadlines.

Chapter 7: Not Scheduling Time to Workout Quotes to Live by

"Everyone has a plan until they get punched in the mouth." – Mike Tyson

"We can make our plans, but it is the Lord who determines our steps." – Proverbs 16:9

"The ultimate inspiration is the deadline." – Nolan Bushnell

"A goal is a dream with a deadline." – Napoleon Hill

"The key is not to prioritize your schedule, but to schedule your priorities." – Steven Covey

Chapter 8: Starting Off With Too Much

Losing weight can be difficult and sometimes overwhelming. At times this is the fault of the person desiring a healthier life. They may be starting out with more than they can handle at the time. The desire is there, but the burden may be too much too soon.

There are skills that need to be mastered to lose weight successfully and keep it off. The learning curve is different for each individual. What one person can handle easily may be a burden for another. One person may be able to handle many different changes in their lifestyle easily. While another can only handle one lifestyle change at a time.

Those that have lost weight successfully have mastered the skills and self-discipline necessary to get results. Yet, there are people who try to lose weight unrealistically quick without mastery of skills and self-discipline. They spend hours at the gym their first day back since last January. They try to lose it all in one day. But, successful weight loss takes time. Starting out with too much too soon can be detrimental to fitness goals.

Storytime: Salt life

When I was working at a nationally-known gym, I was known to kick people out of the gym on their first day. To me, it didn't make sense to not workout for years and try to get it all back on your first day. I have witnessed people spending 4-hours at the gym their first day back. Most people wouldn't understand why I was kicking them out. But I had to make them see that they were sprinting at the beginning of a marathon.

Those that listened to my advice had the energy to come back the next day. Ultimately, they developed consistency through a marathon point-of-view. Those that didn't listen didn't last. They burned themselves out with too much too soon.

There was an overweight gentleman in particular I had to talk off of a treadmill. His first day in, he was on the treadmill for more than an hour. Then I didn't see him for a week. When he came back, I decided to speak to him. He told me that after his first day he had really bad leg cramps for the next several days. I suggested he should start on the bike and work his way up to the treadmill. His body wasn't ready for the intensity yet. He took my advice and I continued to coach him whenever I would see him at the gym.

Initially, he didn't lose much weight but he noticed how his diet would affect his workout. When he ate badly, he worked out badly and would get nauseous. He had a habit of eating takeout or fast-food for most meals in his day. The excess sodium in his diet was so high that you would see the salt on his skin after the workouts. Once he decided to change, everything changed. He got serious about his diet and got rid of the sodium and began losing weight almost immediately. Eventually, he lost over 20 lbs. but most importantly got control of his high blood pressure.

Caught up in the details

There are too many nuances in a healthy lifestyle, especially eating healthy. For example, just eating healthy vs. eating five, small, 300 calorie, gluten-free, organic foods, cooked in extra virgin olive oil. Being too detail-oriented at the beginning can be overwhelming. Someone starting out should be more concerned about mastering the basics before trying something more difficult. If the change requires too much detail or initial effort, it won't last.

There are different levels of mastery to obtain on the road to a healthy lifestyle. Everyone must start at Level-1 before we go to Level-2. However, there are many people who try to start at Level-10 but have not developed the skills and lessons of the previous levels. The technical term is a "shortcut". And with many shortcuts, you will always end up back where you should've started.

With each restart, it becomes harder mentally. This is due to seemingly being at the bottom of the mountain and looking towards the peak. The more you restart, the larger the mountain seems to grow. The climb appears harder as getting the body you want becomes more impossible in your mind. But the truth is the mountain never grew larger. It is still the same mountain. There is still just one way to climb it—one Level at a time.

To elevate through each Level, you have to master the skills at each Level. You practice the skills of that Level until you have mastered it. Practicing the skills consistently develops self-discipline. Eventually, it becomes second nature and you will be prepared to take the test to go to the next Level.

Going to the next Level

Entering the next level is marked with a certain type of adversity or test. You can call it the "Gatekeeper." The ability to overcome the test, or Gatekeeper, signifies that the necessary skills were mastered then access is granted for the next Level for new skills to be learned. This is true. Have you ever noticed that the same issues get in the way every time you try to lose weight? For example: food temptation, family issues, time management, etc. That is because commitment was never mastered at the previous Level.

The same Gatekeeper test will come up each time until you pass the test. If you are always stopped by the same test at the same weight, you have not mastered the necessary skills to pass. When you take a shortcut you are missing out on all the lessons of the previous Levels. Thus, imagine starting off with Level-5 but you have not mastered the skills of Level-1. You don't have the skills necessary to sustain you at Level-5. You will be met with such overwhelming opposition you will burn yourself out. Eventually, you will quit for relief because it becomes too much too soon.

For instance, imagine starting at Level-10 with being perfect with your diet by eating 5 small, gluten-free, whole wheat, organic meals per day. But you have not mastered Level-1 lesson of commitment. The sudden change is not received by your spouse and family. There is instant pushback. Now, to appease them, there need to be two sets of meals prepared for yourself and then your family. This means spending twice as much time and money cooking and preparing foods. In addition, you will have to get up earlier or stay up later to pack your foods for the next day. Also, now there is more stress at work because there is pushback from your co-workers because you are not eating-out with them at lunchtime. Additionally, there is the stress of finding small, perfect, gluten-free, organic alternatives at family events, dinner dates, and late night cravings.

All of this stress doesn't even include exercise. Visualize doing this without mastering commitment, consistency, time management, etc. You are dealing with Level-10 issues with Level 0 skills. No wonder people get overwhelmed and then quit. But this happens every year on January 1st but doesn't even last until January 31st.

The New Year's Resolution pitfalls

Every January, people crowd into gyms all over America in hopes of conquering their New Year's Resolution goals of losing weight. This achievement has escaped them year after year but they begin each year with a new determination. However, this is short-lived. They usually change their diets, begin exercising every day and make other lifestyle changes along with these two major ones.

The "New Year's Resolutionaries" change their sleeping habits getting up earlier to exercise even though they haven't changed going to bed earlier. They change their diet without educating themselves on successful Level-1 changes they need to make. They usually heard from a friend of a friend that lost weight with a certain diet.

At first, it doesn't look like too much because the desire matches the effort. But as the days get longer and the nights get shorter, they run out of energy. Eventually, it gets more and more arduous. It becomes too many changes too soon.

Yet, there are Resolutionaries that are successful at keeping their New Year's Resolutions throughout the year. Their views are more long term than the short-lived Resolutionaries. They do not try to overdo it but begin with what they can commit to. The successful Resolutionaries think progress from where they start and not about getting their goals all at once. The successful start with one weight loss issue at a time and begin mastering that before moving to the next issue. This approach spreads the stress over time so it doesn't become overwhelming. In short, they start small and build from there.

Best Practices: Keep it simple

Because everyone is different, we all have a different Level-1. What you can handle at your Level-1 may be different than what someone else can handle at their Level-1. What is harmful is when we start to compare each other's levels. Therefore, stop comparing yourself to others.

Next, you have to determine what you can be consistent with. This will require that you are completely honest with yourself. If not, you are setting yourself up for failure. You will place more burden than you can currently handle and then eventually quit. Rather, be honest with what you can only handle then begin there. Then focus on developing skills and self-discipline for success at your Level-1.

You must develop skills that will make you more efficient at your current Level. You can only gain mastery of the skill through consistent perfect practice. You are not going to be perfect every day. However, that should not stop you from trying. Practice on being perfect at your level regardless of how you feel that day. There will be challenges with any goal, but you should not let your emotions dictate your actions. If you do, you will get stuck and may never lose weight. Thus, focus on goal attainment through practice, nothing else.

Chapter 8: Starting off With Too Much Quotes to Live by

"You don't have to go fast, you just have to go." – Anonymous

"Make it simple, but significant." – Don Draper

"Our outer world will always be a reflection of our inner world. Our level of success is always going to parallel our level of personal development. Until we dedicate time each day to developing ourselves into the person we need to be to create the life we want, success is always going to be a struggle to attain." – Hal Elrod

"Always bear in mind that your own resolution to succeed is more important than any other." – Abraham Lincoln

"Do not despise these small beginnings, for the Lord rejoices to see the work begin, to see the plumb line in Zerubbabel's hand." – Zechariah 4:10

Chapter 9: Not Being Realistic With Your Diet

Foodies are known for enjoying eating new foods. So much so that it is a hobby for them to seek new foods, tastes, and experiences. Even if you are not a Foodie, food is a large part of everyone's life. Somehow it is always interwoven into our culture through family time, holidays, and celebrations. Even if you are not a Foodie, your diet has to be a large part of your life if you want to lose weight.

The largest part of successfully losing weight is the diet. There is no way for you to lose weight without getting control of your diet. This tends to be the most difficult part of weight loss which is why most people avoid it only to fail at weight loss. Ignoring things won't ever change them- you have to address them. Unfortunately, people are sadly mistaken when they believe they only have to address it once initially and it will fix itself eventually.

Truthfully, gaining control of your diet is a daily task. It is something that must be decided on every morning when you wake up and throughout the day. There will always be weight-gain-opportunities throughout the day. But you decide if you are going to succumb to the temptation or not. Fortunately, if you reject enough weight-gain-opportunities, you will begin losing weight. And more importantly, you will begin forming successful habits for life.

Storytime: A decision to change

There was a training client that I had that was having issues losing weight. At the time I knew why. Even though we would weigh-in monthly and her numbers didn't change. She was always surprised and very disappointed at her weight loss plateau. She was one of the hardest working clients I had. Even though she was overweight, she never allowed that to be an excuse for her effort while working out.

However, I knew until she had the same convictions about her diet she would not lose any weight. She has failed to lose weight for years even though she would try every new diet that came out. Each diet seemed fun at first but unrealistic to maintain. In the end, she would quit and move on to the next diet fad. Thus her results were always inconsistent. Some months she would go up, other months she would go down. One month she made a significant amount of weight loss. But gained it all back and then some within a couple of weeks.

At this point in her life, she wasn't ready for change. She really needed to get serious about her diet if she would ever want to lose weight. After one bad weigh-in, out of frustration, I asked her "What is it going to take for you to finally change?" She was shocked that I asked. She didn't answer but I could tell it made an impact.

The month that she decided to change, she saw her biggest month of weight loss. She has consistently been losing since. This is significant because she has always been an emotional eater. During times of high stress, she would always go to fast-food or high sugary foods for comfort. Afterwards, she would feel bad for quitting on her diet and eat even more as a result.

Her largest weight loss month happened because she stopped dieting altogether. She began a real lifestyle change and got realistic with her diet. She started by incorporating more fruits and vegetables in her diet. She only chose the fruits and vegetables that she liked and expanded from there. She avoided fast food restaurants, which was difficult at first but found healthier alternatives. Last but not least, she found accountability. She joined a support group that really encouraged her and pushed her towards her goals.

Is it worth that slice of cake?

In the beginning levels it is not about being perfect, but improving every single day. Every day you don't improve, you are taking a step back from your goals. No "slice of cake" is worth that. Choosing cake over your fitness goals is a choice to stay fat, unhappy, and uncomfortable in your own skin.

Is the cake really worth it? Short answer: no. No slice of cake is worth being unhappy. But there is a misconception that eating makes people happy. This couldn't be further from the truth. Happiness is a choice. Lasting happiness can never come from outward but only from inward. Thus, no food can make you happy. Great tasting food can be enjoyable but it cannot produce happiness. But, believing that happiness is in food will only deceive you. You will continue overeating in search of happiness but will never find it. Don't mistake being full or satiated with happiness.

That faux happiness is fleeting. Once the cake is gone, so will your happiness. Then you have to refill your happiness with another slice of cake. But if you choose to be happy regardless of your circumstance, you will find true happiness. Then you will discover the inner strength needed to pursue your goals.

Seeing weight loss results will encourage you to continue to press towards your goals. There is nothing more satisfying than putting in the work and seeing inches fall off or the number on the scale decreasing. Nothing will make you happier than having self-confidence. Therefore, choose results over cake.

Eating your way to weight loss

Drastic changes to anyone's diet may not work. It may have an initial impact but it isn't lasting because it may be too difficult to stick to. A better approach may be to find a way of incorporating healthy foods, which you should be eating, into your diet like fruits, vegetables, and water. Then you should slowly increase the intake of the healthy foods. Eventually, you will crave the unhealthy foods less. This proven approach allows you to slowly and successfully ween off of bad foods.

This strategy keeps you from feeling deprived and focusing on what you can't have. The depriving feeling is one of the main reasons why most people quit diets. Essentially, this is why restrictive diets don't work long-term. Restrictive or crash diets cut large amounts of calories out of a healthy daily intake for quick weight loss results. They do produce results; however, they are short-lived because the restrictions are unrealistic and impossible to stick to long-term. In the short-term, you will lose 10 lbs., but eventually gain 15 lbs. back from binging on the foods you were deprived of.

This is known as Yo-yo Dieting, which is the cycle many crash dieters are on. These dieters want to lose weight, but they keep gaining the weight back as a result of the binge eating after quick weight loss success. Losing weight and keeping it off is a slower process. There are skills to master to keep the weight off long term and they cannot be overlooked. More importantly, there are food issues that need to be unlearned. Incorporating more fruits, vegetables, and water allows you to lose weight while learning the healthy habits and unlearning the unhealthy ones. With a realistic diet, you will lose weight, but more importantly, you will prevent yo-yo dieting weight gain.

Food is fuel

Another change that needs to be made for weight loss success is Food-Perspective. Only seeing food as pleasure can be a hindrance to weight loss success. Perspective determines behavior. The fattest people on the planet don't have the same view of food as the fittest people on the planet. Fat people see food as pleasure while fit people see food as fuel for their bodies. And the two views are significantly different and worth pointing out the difference.

Here are some of the differences with fat people. The fattest people on the planet see unhealthy food as pleasure and have a negative view of healthy food. They tend to involve unhealthy food into different aspects of their lives. For example, unhealthy food must be present while spending time with friends and family. They attribute the food to having more fun at family events. Unhappiness in their lives tends to lead them to emotional eating. Their mood dictates how much junk food they will eat. The junk food leads to low energy which leads to low activity and more weight gain.

However, the fittest people on the planet have a different view of food. Food is fuel. They are worried about eating the right types of foods to fuel their next workout. Eating high-energy foods gives them the energy to stay active and chase their goals in all areas of their lives. They maintain high energy which keeps them from emotional eating. Junk food is seen as food for special events and in moderation only. They understand how junk food saps their energy and abstain from it. They tend to do more active activities with their friends and family rather than sitting and eating. Because they are fitter and have the energy, they are able to enjoy other aspects of life outside of food.

Changing your food-perspective will take time. Having a healthier food-perspective can lead to more energy and a higher sense of well-being. Unhealthy eating will only lead to more unhealthy eating and weight gain. But, as you increase the amounts of healthy foods you will notice the difference in energy and your ability to do more active undertakings. But more importantly, you will notice the difference on how food affects your mood.

Best practices: Changing your food mindset

The first step is to decide to be happy. I know this does not sound like a health and fitness advice but deciding to be happy puts you in control of your emotions rather than allow circumstances to control your emotions. Gaining control over your emotions empowers you. Happiness becomes internal rather than external. Once you realize that, you are able to separate food from your happiness. Therefore, wake up every morning and decide whatever happens you will be happy.

The second step is to find healthier alternatives than eating to relieve stress. Because there will be high-stressed days that will challenge your commitment to being healthy. If you don't have healthy channels to relieve the stress, you will revert back to eating for happiness. Therefore, you have to find a healthier way to relieve the stress like exercise, dancing to your favorite album, biking, or walking.

The third step is to find healthy activities to do with friends and family. Begin a healthy tradition with family by finding creative ways to stay active during gatherings. For example, suggest going bowling or ice skating for birthdays instead of having a traditional house party. By substituting the activities with your family and friends, you will be focused on developing those relationships and less on food.

The final step is avoiding situations that may compromise your commitment to yourself and your diet. This may include spending time with friends and family that do not share your new interest in becoming healthy. Don't avoid them completely, but avoid situations where you are unable to say no to unhealthy temptation.

Changing your food-perspective will take time. It never happens overnight. Only with practice and time will it become a healthy lifelong habit.

Chapter 9: Not Being Realistic With Your Diet Quotes to Live by

"The way we see the world creates the world we see." – Barry Neil Kaufman

"As a man thinks in his heart so is he." – Proverbs 23: 7

"The secret of change is to focus all of your energy not on fighting the old but on building the new." – Socrates

"Nothing tastes as good as skinny feels." – Anonymous

"If food is your best friend, then it is also your worst enemy." –Anonymous

Chapter 10: Giving Up Too Soon

It is always too early to quit. If losing weight is something that you deeply desire, then you have to be willing to do what it takes to achieve it. It won't be easy. And it will only come with a lot of sacrifices, but it will be worth it. However, believing that any goal is achievable without opposition is unrealistic. Adversity is part of the process, it comes at every level. But if you don't believe you have what it takes to endure the challenges and overcome, then you are already defeated.

Don't give up too soon. You have to be single-minded when it comes to achieving your goals. You can't be focused on anything else because what you focus on magnifies. Thus, you have to win in your mind before you win anywhere else.

Mind War

The battle that must be won is in the mind. Hence, if you are defeated in your mind, you will be defeated in life. This only makes sense if you look back on your own experiences as proof. When you were ready to quit chasing a goal, what was the conversation like in your head? Was it all empowering and confident? Or, was the conversation condemning and magnifying the difficulties? In my experiences, the difference in the conversation is always the difference in winning and losing the battle in the mind.

In the past, during the times of conquest, when a kingdom defeated another kingdom in war, the losers were forced to become slaves and subjects of the victors. Most times, the winning kingdom would place soldiers and leaders to govern the conquered people. The losing kingdom would stay as slaves and subjects to the conquering kingdom until they were fed up with being slaves and subjects. Their desire for liberty had to be greater than their fear as slaves and subjects.

This is also true in Mind Wars. When you quit, you become a slave to weight loss. You will always think that the difficulties in losing weight will always be greater than you. Too great to overcome. Too great for you to ever attain your weight loss goals. You will find yourself avoiding the subject of losing weight more and more. You will feel like a quitter and will be known as a quitter to yourself and others.

Waking up your Inner Conqueror

But, in the past, during times of conquest, once the slaves and subjects were fed up with being slaves, they found the courage to be free. The slaves and subjects would lead a revolt against the conquering kingdom and fight for their freedom. Throughout history, it wasn't the kingdom with the best army that won, but the kingdom that was willing to do whatever it took to win.

The same is true in life; once you are fed up with quitting, fed up with losing, and fed up with being unhappy, you are ready for victory. You will find the courage once you are ready to do whatever it takes to win. No Plan-B, just you achieving your main goal. You will awaken your Inner-Conqueror. Your desire fuels your Inner-Conqueror to overcome your challenges and realize your dreams. You have the capability of defeating weight loss once and for all. But, your dream needs you to endure the adversity and challenges to finally breakthrough. You cannot quit too early otherwise, you will never have victory.

There are many people who had success losing weight. But there is nothing greater in them than what lies dormant within you. In previous chapters, I spoke about how adversity pulls out what is in us—our Inner-Conqueror. The nature of our Inner-Conqueror is to overcome. Drawing it out takes the courage to endure even when you don't see any results. The longer we stay in the fight, the stronger we can become. But quitting only makes us weak.

Most people that have successfully lost weight and kept it off only did so after failing several times. They tried and failed but they kept trying. They all started new diets and quit their new diets. They have all had setbacks. They had good days and really bad days. However, it wasn't until they were fed up that they awoke their Inner-Conqueror. Their Inner-Conqueror kept them going during the difficult times when it seemed like there was no way for them to succeed. But they chose to be uncomfortable and push towards their dreams rather than quitting. They needed to realize that their challenges were all part of the process and they needed to withstand them to breakthrough. Their Inner-Conqueror would not allow any obstacle to get in their way; instead, they decided to double-down to reach victory.

Storytime: The power of a made-up mind

In 1519, the great Spanish Conquistador (conqueror), Hernan Cortes, landed on the beaches of Veracruz (present day: Mexico) with the hopes of great conquest against the Aztecs. His men were fearful of the battle ahead and their murmuring eventually reached the ear of Cortes. Hearing this, Cortes knew that given the opportunity, his men would desert him if faced with any adversity. Therefore, he ordered that the ships be burned leaving no way for retreat. Afterwards, they pursued the conquest of the Aztecs. They eventually defeated the multitude of Aztec warriors in battle with only 600 Spaniards and the help of another local tribe.

When you are fed up, you don't have room for quit. Refuse to lose, and fight your way to victory. The Conquistadors burned their ships for victory. Would you be willing to do the same? Are you willing to awaken your Inner-Conqueror by pushing yourself further than you ever have before? On the other side of your obstacle is the realization of your dream. But, you have to be willing to fight your way through it to attain your weight loss goals.

Best Practices: Developing a Victor's Mindset

The victory begins in the mind. But it takes time to develop grit, or the mindset to never quit. Firstly, the most difficult thing to do is change the inner conversation. What are you saying to yourself over and over? If there was someone following you around saying the negative comments you say to yourself, you wouldn't wait too long before you tell them "where to go." Yet, why do we speak so negatively to ourselves?

There are only a few seconds before a thought takes root and grows within the mind. Get in the practice of paying attention to your thoughts. You have the power to stop a thought, reject it, and then replace it with a positive affirming thought. Though you cannot stop a negative thought from entering your mind, you do have the choice to accept the thought or reject it. Thus, every negative thought that goes against you and your goals must be rejected. Then repeat the positive affirmation of your strength, ability and commitment to achieve your goals to yourself over and over again. For example, "I can do this" or "I will succeed." Repeating the positive affirmations increases the subconscious belief in what is said. The same is also true for negative declarations like "I can't" or "it's too hard." Changing negative thought patterns to more positive ones takes time and much practice. But in time, it will become easier until it becomes a permanent behavior.

Secondly, you have to immerse yourself in a positive culture. Remember, like learning a new language, it is easier if you immerse yourself into the culture. This means that you cannot be around negativity whatsoever. This includes negative people, negative images, and negative sounds. Our environment has an immense influence on our beliefs, attitudes, and behaviors. You will be surprised what negativity we allow into our environment that affects our self-image, self-esteem, and self-confidence. Simple things like what we watch on television, listen to in our cars, negative people at work or at home. All are influencing us negatively. Some of the most successful people on the planet isolate themselves from all negativity. They engross themselves in an environment of positivity. They avoid anything that isn't building them up and pushing them towards their dreams. Think about how Olympic athletes are trained in isolation to achieve world-class goals. They are only around team coaches and trainers most of the day. Their team is meant to perfect them and help build them up mentally and physically. You may not be able to train in isolation like Olympic athletes, but you do have control over your environment. You can build your own team of coaches and trainers with technology that we have today.

Your mind is your kingdom, you have to be vigilant in guarding your mind against intruders. You have to guard against negativity. One way to supercharge your mind is having an early morning routine. It has to be done daily for it to work. I encourage you to try it for 21 days and watch your mindset shift like never before.

21-Day Challenge

The first step is getting up early enough to have time to do it. Yes, this will require getting up 30-45 minutes earlier than usual. Once you get up, read your goals aloud to yourself in the positive past-tense affirmation like you have already achieved it. For example, "I lost 20 lbs. by (insert date)." Afterwards, you begin listening to positive motivational podcast, motivational YouTube videos, or sermon while you are getting ready. Then read for 15-minutes in a personal development book of your choice. Eat breakfast in silence and meditate on what you have to accomplish that day. See yourself already achieving that goal. Then, in your car, listen to an audiobook or podcast on the area you want to improve in. While at work, only listen to positive upbeat music.

In 21-days you will notice a shift in your mindset. The negativity in your environment that went unnoticed will irk you to the point of removing it out of your environment. You will want to do more things that build you up rather than tear you down. Then after doing it for 21-days straight, challenge yourself to do the same for 21-days both before work and after work. After work, drive home listening to an audiobook. At home, listen to a sermon, motivation podcast, or motivational YouTube video as you unwind for the day. Avoid watching mindless television and instead, read a book on personal development. Take time to do more active things with your family like going for a walk or going to the park.

It will be difficult and will take time to replace these negative influences with more positive ones; however, it will be worth it. You know that you have achieved this second step when you find yourself unable to be around any kind of negativity. You will avoid negative people. You will avoid negative images. And you will begin noticing all the negative words that enter your environment. You won't allow the negativity to stay.

In closing

You can only become unstoppable if you decide not to stop. Burn your boats and double-down when you are met with adversity. If you believe in yourself, then you will achieve any dream. This book is meant to be put into practice not just to be read through cover to cover.

This book was written for the purpose of building a successful mindset. I didn't want it to be just another health or fitness book. For this book to be helpful, it had to work on the person from the inside-out. For the change to last, it has to occur inwardly first. What shows on the outside usually is an indication of what is going on internally. Therefore, if there is a lack of success with a healthy diet and exercise, there is some deficiency inwardly. This book was meant to address the deficiency in a practical way.

Most gyms will work on you from the outside-in. They don't really address what is going on inwardly. They expect the exercise to fix everything. It doesn't always work out like that. If you teach people how to empower themselves there is no telling what they will be able to achieve.

I repeated a lot of the same principles throughout the book on purpose. Repetition is the best way to learn. Once you hear the thought over and over again, you will internalize it. Once it begins to annoy you, then you know you have internalized and will never forget it. It will be there for you in times of adversity, pulling you towards your goal. It will allow you to ignore your emotions and focus on the promise behind the principle. As long as you endure, you will reap the promise of the principle.

Be encouraged. You can achieve your weight loss goals. Choose today that you won't be stopped. Choose today that you will achieve your goal no matter what. Then you will realize it is only time that is between you and your goal.

Chapter 10: Giving Up Too Soon Quotes to Live by

"It's always too early to quit." – Norman Vincent Peale

"Failure doesn't come from falling down, failure comes from not getting back up." –Anonymous

"I can do all things through Christ who strengthens me." – Philippians 4:13

"It all begins and ends in your mind, what you give power to has power over you, if you allow it." – Leon Brown

"There is nothing more powerful than the made-up mind." —Lewis Gordon Pugh

About The Author

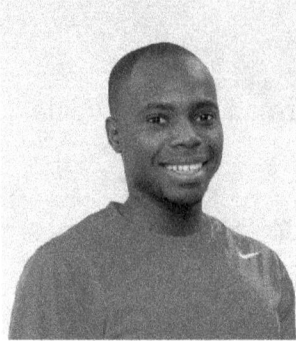

Gladimir Simeon, B.S.

Health Fitness Specialist

You <u>know</u> you have it in you to change.

But do you <u>believe</u> you can change?

Gladimir "Coach Glad" Simeon, founder of Glad Health & Fitness, is an experienced fitness expert, dynamic speaker and fitness trainer who educates and empowers his diverse clientele to conquer personal and physical challenges.

Glad goes beyond the tips and quick-fix gimmicks seen in the media and understands that in order to achieve success in all areas of life, mental hurdles must first be overcome.

Through his knowledgeable, humorous and intuitive approach, negative thinking is redirected into positive thinking. It is one thing to know but it is another to believe you have it in you to change. Harness your internal strength to transform your external circumstances.

Gladimir Simeon earned his Bachelor of Science degree in Exercise Science and Health Promotion from Florida Atlantic University in the hope of enriching people's lives through fitness.

A Call to Purpose

Since its inception in February 2010, Glad felt the need to do more with his company to reach people in need. After working in a gym of a well-known national fitness company, he realized that he was limited to what he could do to help clients. He soon realized that they needed more than what a typical gym could offer them. Many people come to gyms looking for support for their health and fitness, but these facilities lack the comprehensive approach necessary to help with long-term weight loss.

In September 2012, Gladimir began changing the structure of his company to better serve the masses. A change was needed in the health and fitness industry. The need for change garnered the unique approach of Glad Health & Fitness—lasting change from the inside-out. The launching of our Wellness Expansion Programs soon followed. Now Glad Health & Fitness is on a mission to change industry standards. We believe you have it in you to change and our programs will prove it to you.